Meriam Khadhar

Teaching from the patient management problem:

Meriam Khadhar

Teaching from the patient management problem:

how about learning by playing?

ScienciaScripts

Imprint

Cover image: www.ingimage.com

This book is a translation from the original published under ISBN 978-620-6-72365-3.

Publisher:
Sciencia Scripts
is a trademark of
Dodo Books Indian Ocean Ltd. and OmniScriptum S.R.L publishing group

120 High Road, East Finchley, London, N2 9ED, United Kingdom
Str. Armeneasca 28/1, office 1, Chisinau MD-2012, Republic of Moldova, Europe
Printed at: see last page
ISBN: 978-620-8-28041-3

CHAPTER 1

The issue of medical training is a topic of discussion in all medical faculties. As teachers, we have a responsibility to ensure an effective learning process by providing a high level of theoretical teaching in small groups and by offering practical training at appropriate training sites, in accordance with the reform plan that was put in place back in 1988 [1].

The modern pedagogical approach has considerably transformed the role of the teacher, who no longer confines himself to imparting knowledge, but must now actively support the learner in the autonomous acquisition of his knowledge.

The Patient Management Problem (PMP) is an innovative teaching method based on contextualised learning and teaching to assess clinical reasoning.

Since its creation in the 1960s [2], the "Patient Management Problem" (PMP) has been widely used in learning and also in the evaluation of initial and postgraduate medical studies. However, in Tunisia, its use remains very limited. Few studies have been carried out to assess how learners view this type of learning. The student assigned to the Nephrology Department at the Mongi Slim Hospital in La Marsa took part in a PMP-type tutorial session. However, this teaching was not evaluated.

The aim of this study was :

- To evaluate directed teaching in the form of PMP as a means of learning clinical reasoning in second-year medical students and, more specifically, in the management of hyperkalaemia in specific situations.

- To assess learners' perceptions of the value of the PMP as a means of learning or assessment in nephrology.

The results of this study could have important implications for medical education and could help to improve the learning of clinical skills among future doctors.

CHAPTER 2

1. Type of study :

We carried out a descriptive cross-sectional study, which included 6 "PMP" type directed teaching sessions (DE) in Nephrology, which took place in the field.

2. Study population :

- Inclusion criteria: All second-year students in the second cycle of medical studies (DCEM2) assigned to the nephrology rotation at the Mongi Slim la Marsa Hospital during the second semester of the 2022-2023 academic year were included.

- Exclusion criteria: All learners who did not attend the DE (absent or excluded following a mark in the pre-requisite test < 4/10) were excluded.

- We carried out a total of six sessions with 5 to 7 learners per group. The study included a total of 30 day students. Thirty-four students were assigned to our department by the faculty in the second semester of 2023, but four learners were absent. No learner was excluded because of an eliminatory mark in the pre-test.

3. Directed teaching tools: the Patient Management Problem

By clicking on each proposal, a hypertext link was sent to a slide containing the expected response to this choice, the rating awarded and a commentary. To calculate the PMP score, we used the scoring scale used at the Tunis Faculty of Medicine (3), giving a positive score (+1 or +2) to proposals considered useful or essential, and a zero or negative score to proposals considered useless or dangerous for the patient. Correct answers that were not chosen in the correct order were given a score of 0. Two propositions risked jeopardising the patient's vital prognosis, in which case the test was interrupted. The learner in this case received a mark of zero.

4. Planning the session :

4.1. Theme of the tutorial sessions :

The topic covered during this PMP was the management of hyperkalaemia. This topic was one of the educational objectives for medical students and we chose it because of its relevance, its seriousness and the need for urgent management of this type of situation. The case we proposed was illustrated by a real observation.

It is important for GPs to be able to provide urgent care before referring patients to a nephrologist. Learners were informed of the subject before the course and the programme was posted in the staff room at the start of the course.

4.2. Preparing the Patient Management Problem :

The PMP was written by the session monitor (myself) with reference to an actual patient file. It was in electronic format (Microsoft Powerpoint® version 16.72). The first slide of the PMP contained the clinical vignette, followed by an instruction slide which also explained the PMP scoring scale, and then a slide with a list of 12 proposals to choose from.

4.3. Pre-test preparation :

The pre-test consisted of MCQs, ROCQs and a clinical case (appendix 1) and lasted 10 minutes. The mark awarded was out of 10. This gave an initial mark. In addition, the learner should be excluded if he/she had a mark < 4/10.

5. Course of the session :

The sessions took place in the staff room. Each session lasted between 100 and 130 minutes. The session began with a briefing lasting 10 to

15 minutes, during which the teacher presented the general framework of the session and the steps involved in carrying it out, and explained how the PMP worked to the learners. The students then took the pre-test individually, which lasted 10 minutes per student. The session was ended with a 20-minute group debriefing, followed by the post-test and satisfaction questionnaire.

6. Evaluation of teaching: (assessment criteria)

The final mark was determined on the basis of the score obtained out of 20 points. To assess knowledge, answer sheets filled in by learners during guided teaching sessions were distributed and then analysed.

Immediate educational effectiveness was analysed on the basis of two main criteria: cognitive gain and degree of satisfaction.

Theoretical knowledge was assessed using a knowledge questionnaire before (pre-test: appendix 1) and at the end (post-test: appendix 1) of each DE session. Learner satisfaction data was collected using an opinion questionnaire on the course and the value of the teaching (appendix 2).

7. Data collection and analysis:

Pre-tests, post-tests and opinion questionnaires were collected and corrected. Marks were awarded to each student according to their performance. Each answer to a question was scored according to its correctness (0 for a wrong answer, 0.5 for an incomplete answer and 1 for a correct answer). The 5-level non-metric ordinal Likert scale was used to analyse the opinion questionnaire. The open-ended comments on this questionnaire were also analysed.

8. Analysis statistics

The data collected was processed using Excel 2013 for data entry and SPSS 20.0 for statistical analysis. Qualitative variables were presented as absolute and relative frequencies (in percentages), while quantitative variables were expressed as means, standard deviations and extreme values.

9. Bibliographic research :

The bibliographical search was carried out using search engines such as "Pub Med" and "Science direct", using the following key words: learning, clinical reasoning, PMP (patient management problem), Evaluation. We are only interested in publications in French and

English.

1O. Ethical considerations :

There was no conflict of interest.

All the learners gave their consent and were aware that the results of the knowledge and satisfaction tests would be used for scientific purposes, but anonymously.

CHAPTER 3

1. Learner characteristics and teaching sessions

The number of learners who took part in the PMP was 30, 23 women and 7 men. Four learners were excluded for absence. No student scored less than 4 out of 10 in the pre-requisite test. Fifteen learners have already had PMP sessions in other speciality departments other than nephrology.

2. Results of the patient management problem :

Taking all learners together, 83.3% passed the PMP assessment. The average mark was 11.11 ± 5.67, with extremes of 0 and 18.46/20. Five students scored zero because they had chosen the proposal that led to the patient's death.

3. Pre- and post-test results :

All thirty learners who took part obtained scores above the pre-set threshold. The average pre-test score was 6.6/10 and the average post-test score was 9.03/10. The scores are summarised in Figure 1

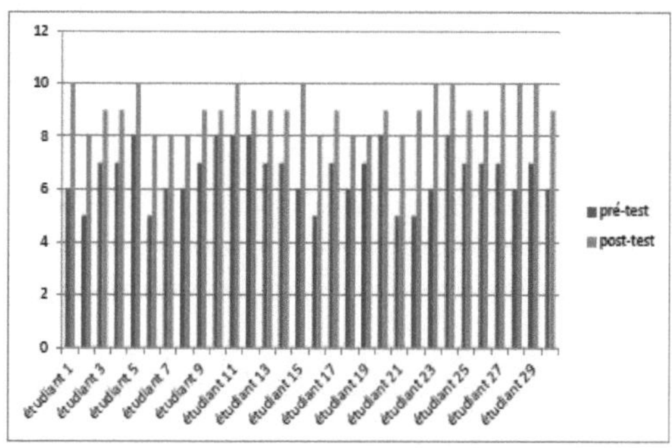

Figure 1: Variations in pre- and post-test scores

4. Gain cognitive

The improvement in learners' average scores was 2.43 [1-4] The improvement in learners' scores (post-test score - pre-test score) is shown in Figure 2.

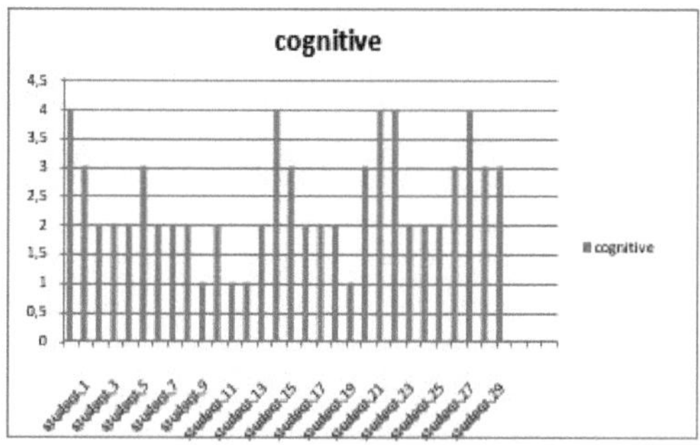

Figure 2: Cognitive gain

4.1. Results of the Patient Management Problem satisfaction questionnaire

4.2. Learners' previous experience with the Patient Management Problem :

Fifteen learners (50%) had already had an apprenticeship with the PMP: thirteen during the DCEM2 paediatrics placement and two during the neonatology placement in the same year 2022-2023. Of these students, three were very satisfied with this learning, four fairly satisfied, six fairly dissatisfied and two very dissatisfied. With regard to assessment by the PMP, only five learners had already had it during the paediatric ECOSMs in DCEM2. One of them was very satisfied, one fairly satisfied, two fairly dissatisfied and one very dissatisfied. These learners stated that the of these PMPs was different from that of the current session, in particular due to the absence of feedback.

4.3. Evaluation of the Patient Management Problem session by the learners :

Thirty opinion questionnaires were completed by learners after the PMP session. In our study, we took a number of factors into account to assess learners' opinions, including the time allocated to the session, skills acquisition, whether or not the PMP was recommended as a means of learning and assessment in SMCEs, and the stress that the PMP may cause learners. The majority of students 'agreed' or 'strongly agreed' with the elements assessed by the opinion questionnaire All learners felt that the time allocated to the session was very consistent; well split between the briefing, the test and the debrief. Ninety per cent of learners felt that the PMP was a useful learning tool that would change the way they think and they agreed that it should be used regularly in teaching. Eighty percent of learners thought that the PMP was better than the 76.6% were in favour of its regular use during SMCEs, but 66.6% of learners found the PMP a stressful means of assessment. Learners' responses to the opinion questionnaire on the session "Management of threatening hyperkalaemia in chronic dialysis patients" are reported in Figure 3.

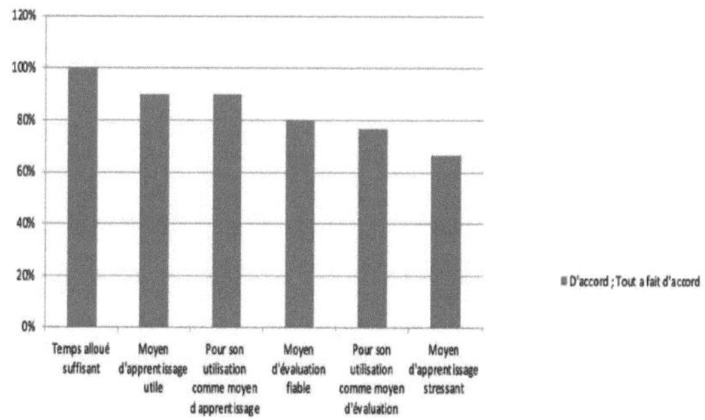

Figure 3: Learners' responses to the opinion questionnaire

4.4. Results of open comments

Of the 30 satisfaction questionnaire forms, 5 contained free comments, as follows:

- The pmp is very interesting but stressful

- The PMP is difficult to use as an assessment tool because it is stressful.

- Very interesting session but we also want the topos

- Very interesting session. We look forward to more PMP sessions.

- Thank you for this PMP on would have liked to have this kind of teaching in all subjects.

CHAPTER 4

The aim of this cross-sectional and descriptive study was to evaluate the impact of directed teaching, in the form of PMP, on the learning of clinical reasoning. It involved 30 second-year medical students assigned to the Nephrology Department of the Mongi Slim Hospital in La Marsa during the second semester of 2023. We proposed a PMP session on the management of hyperkalaemia in a specific situation for each group.

The results of this study indicated a clear improvement in the cognitive performance of the participants, as evidenced by the significant increase in the average score between the pre- and post-test, rising from 6.9 to 9.03/10. Students also expressed a high level of satisfaction with the teaching sessions, describing their effectiveness in helping them to better understand the course. Ninety percent of students felt that these sessions contributed positively to their ability to solve problems. These results attest to the effectiveness of this teaching method.

Weaknesses and strengths of our study :

Some positive aspects of the situation should be noted:

-This is the first experience of using PMP as a learning method in the nephrology section.

-The aim of the study was to evaluate the PMP as a means of learning by assessing the cognitive gain as well as the satisfaction of the learners.

- The subject addressed by the PMP, hyperkalaemia, is a relevant one given its seriousness, and it is a chapter that must be well mastered by the family doctor.

However, our study has certain limitations:

- Firstly, the number of participants in the study was limited, with only 34 learners, four of whom were absent. These students were assigned by the placements department.

- The PMP was of a purely therapeutic nature, and the diagnostic part was not addressed.

1. Guided teaching tools: the Patient Management Problem

Among the various methods for learning and assessing clinical reasoning, the PMP is considered to be an effective method for promoting clinical reasoning and decision-making [3].

Tl was developed in the United States in the mid-1960s [2]. Since then, it has been widely used for learning and evaluation of initial and postgraduate medical studies. In Tunisia, its use remains limited in current practice, although there is a seminar at the Tunis Faculty of Medicine (FMT) on the design and implementation of PMPs. The PMP confronts the learner with a clinical problem to be solved [4]. This method encourages an evolutionary approach to problem-solving that does not rely solely on theoretical knowledge, because of a particular context. In this way, the PMP focuses more on the intellectual process of reasoning than simply on memorising knowledge.

2. Assessment of supervised teaching :

2.1. Definition and general information:

Assessment involves gathering relevant, valid and reliable information. It is an essential part of the teaching-learning process, as it enables us to analyse the knowledge acquired, identify gaps and measure learners' progress by determining whether learning objectives have been achieved [5].

Students receive feedback on their knowledge, skills and learning strategies [6-9].

Evaluation also allows us to gather information on the effectiveness of teaching tools, so that we can make improvements for the future.

It is therefore important to plan the evaluation from the outset [10].

2.2. Assessment procedures :

Assessment is divided into two types: summative and formative.

Summative assessment is used to measure the knowledge and skills acquired at the end of a course or learning period. It is used to make a final decision on the learner's success or failure. Formative assessment is used to provide feedback to students throughout the learning process. It identifies the student's strengths and weaknesses and provides advice on how to improve performance. Formative assessment is often used to help students achieve their learning objectives and improve their understanding of the subjects studied. It provides both the learner and the teacher with objective information about the nature and quality of the learning taking place [9].

There are various models of training evaluation, each with its own advantages and limitations. [11]. Here are a few examples:

- Kirkpatrick model: Tl was developed in 1959. This model is one of the most widely used in training evaluation. Tl has four levels:

reaction, learning, behaviour and results (Figure 5). Tl makes it possible to measure the effectiveness of training at different levels. [5].

- CTPP model: This model focuses on the four key elements of training evaluation: context, input, process and output. It makes it possible to analyse each stage of the training process and identify strengths and weaknesses. [12-14].

It is important to choose the most appropriate training evaluation model according to the specific objectives and needs of the organisation or educational institution.

The different levels of assessment must be put in place in a precise order because there is a causal link between each level. Thus, adequate satisfaction is necessary for effective learning, quality learning is necessary for successful transfer of skills, and successful transfer is necessary to obtain good results. In addition, the higher the level of evaluation, the more important the information gathered is for the institution. [5].

In our study, we chose to set up a formative evaluation project. The evaluation focused on Kirkpatrick's second level, which aims to measure learning outcomes beyond simple learner satisfaction. This level focuses on measuring the skills, knowledge or behaviours acquired as a result of the training. The most direct way of measuring these results is to test the acquisition of new skills in relation to the training objectives. Our aim is not to punish external learners, but rather to support them in their training by providing them with constructive feedback.

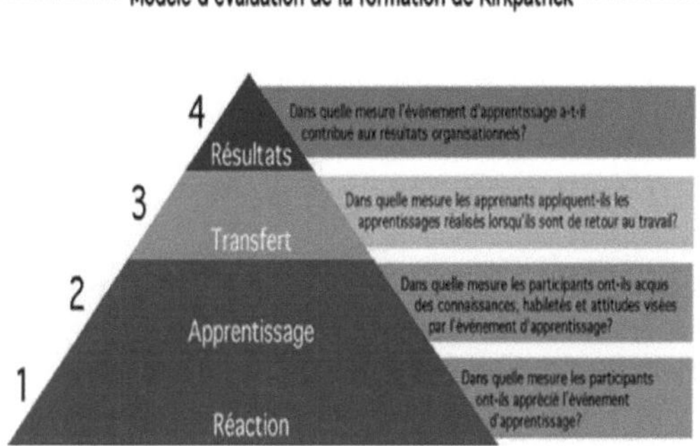

Figure 4: Evaluation of a training course using Kirkpartick's model

2.3. Pre-test - post-test :

"The purpose of the pre-test is to check that the learner has a minimum level of knowledge that will enable him or her to participate effectively in the exercise. So there is no risk of wasting their time or that of their classmates". [1].

A minimum score of 40% (4/10) is required in the pre-test to allow the learner to attend the training session. If this is not the case, the student must return to the patients to resume their training activities [1].

In our study, the placement periods did not always coincide with the theoretical courses given at the faculty. Only 3 out of 6 groups had already attended nephrology courses at the faculty before or during their placement with the service. For this reason, we ensured that learners were informed in advance of the topics to be covered in order to prepare them as well as possible. The pre-test consisted of multiple-choice questions (MCQs), open-ended questions and a clinical case. No student was excluded from the study for a mark of less than 4. Four externs were absent. We reused the same assessment for the post-test at the end of the training.

The post-test is used to measure a learner's level of understanding or mastery of the subject after a period of teaching or training [15].

By comparing the results of the post-test and the pre-test, we can determine the effectiveness of the teaching by measuring the improvement in the learner's knowledge or skills. [16].

2.4. Satisfaction questionnaire for Patient Management Problem sessions:

We set up a questionnaire at the end of each session to obtain feedback from learners on the teaching provided using a PMP.

This evaluation made it possible to measure the level of satisfaction of the learners (Kirkpatrick level 1). The students appreciated the teaching method, finding it useful for assimilating the course and learning to reason. clinical. These results are in line with those reported in the literature, where the majority of learners appreciate this type of teaching and consider it beneficial for their learning and exam preparation [17-18].

In our study, learners responded positively to the process, content and pedagogical method used for PMP-based directed learning. They also suggested that other sessions of this type of teaching should be held and that this method should be generalised during subsequent placements in nephrology and other specialities. These suggestions motivate us to prepare and carry out other PMP sessions. Our results are in line with the literature, which shows that learners prefer active learning methods, such as problem solving or clinical case studies, rather than traditional methods based on simple memorization [19-20].

Although the evaluation of learner satisfaction is an interesting criterion, it is not sufficient to evaluate the effectiveness of teaching [21].

3.Cognitive gain :

Our study revealed that the PMP led to a significant cognitive gain, as shown by the results of the pre-test and post-test. All learners acquired new knowledge, whatever their starting level. Several studies have highlighted the value of using the PMP in medical education, both for the initial training of medical students [3, 10] and for the continuing education of practitioners [4].Marquis et al demonstrated that a self-teaching programme including three PMPs led to a significant improvement in knowledge among GPs. Moreover, according to the learners' comments, three quarters of the knowledge acquired was used in their current practice [4].Afroza et al conducted a comparative study in paediatrics between a conventional teaching programme and a Problem-based Learning (PBL) teaching programme, which included 25 PMPs [22]. They subsequently carried out an evaluation by ECOSM and concluded that PMP learning was more effective than conventional teaching.Results from the Golchai et al study showed that over 80% of midwives who had undertaken learning about gestational diabetes through a PMP reported that it had been beneficial to the development of their clinical reasoning and decision making [3].In ben Abdelaziz's study, they observed a significant improvement in students' marks at post-test, regardless of the type of test. This suggests that the PMP is an effective learning tool [23].

4. Feedback from learners :

In terms of feedback from our students, the PMP was well appreciated. The majority were in favour of using it regularly for learning and assessment. This reinforces the idea that the PMP can be an effective teaching and assessment method in healthcare. In our study, we found that two-thirds of students found the PMP stressful because of the presentation in solo in front of the tutor. We found no studies specifically assessing learners' perception of stress when using the PMP method for teaching or assessment.

5. Practical recommendations and future prospects :

This work enabled us to estimate the educational effectiveness of the PMP as a method of learning clinical reasoning. Despite the small number of students, it appears that directed teaching using a PMP is an appreciated and useful learning method, since it seems to have facilitated our students' learning. However, further studies would be needed to assess the change in practical behaviour over the longer term, since the immediate impact on knowledge is not necessarily correlated with an impact on practical performance [24,25].We have observed that the use of PMP in the Faculty of Medicine in Tunis remains very limited in practice for learning and assessment. This may be due to factors such as the time required to design, validate and produce PMPs, a lack of experience and training in this teaching tool on the part of teachers, and the need for certain computer skills [26,27]. Producing a complete PMP requires a significant investment on the part of the trainer to be able to choose the right theme, method and prepositions [4]

For the future, we propose to :

- To promote the production and validation of several PMPs within the Nephrology Section and to create a database containing at least two PMPs for each pathology listed in the DCEM2 externship logbook (one for the formative evaluation and the other for the ECOSM).

- Generalise the PMP as a means of learning from the first practical training courses, with the following objectives well-defined educational programmes and standardised planning across the various training sites.

- Incorporate the PMP into all MSCE tests and clinical examinations.

CHAPTER 5

The PMP is a teaching tool developed in the United States in the mid-1960s. Since then, it has been widely used for learning and assessment in initial and postgraduate medical studies. In Tunisia, its use remains very limited. The aim of this study was to evaluate the impact of learning using the PMP in practical nephrology teaching, as well as learners' perceptions of the value of the PMP in learning and assessment. We conducted a prospective evaluative study in the nephrology department of the Mongi Slim Hospital in La Marsa. We included DCEM2 students on nephrology placements who were willing to take part. We prepared a PMP in electronic format on the management of threatening hyperkalaemia in the chronic haemodialysis patient. The PMP began with a clinical label slide, followed by an instructions slide that also explained the PMP scoring scale, and then a slide with a list of 20 proposals to choose from. Each proposal was hyperlinked to a slide containing the expected response to that choice and a comment if necessary. To calculate the PMP score, we used the rating scale in use at the Tunis Faculty of Medicine. To assess the students' knowledge, we used tests comprising MCQ, QROC and other questions. and a level 2 and 3 QROC clinical case answering the following questions same PMP learning objectives. The same test was used as a pre- and post-test. A questionnaire was prepared to assess learners' level of satisfaction after the learning session. Responses to the evaluation questions were scored using a Liekert scale. The teaching session included a briefing phase, followed by the pre-test, the PMP session carried out individually, the group debriefing phase, the post-test and the satisfaction questionnaire.Thirty students took part in the study. All students combined, 83% achieved an average score in the PMP assessment.

The PMP led to a significant improvement in the assessment test scores and consequently to the acquisition of new knowledge. All students combined, the post-test scores (9.03) were higher than those for the pre-test (6.6). This improvement was observed regardless of the learners' starting level. Fifteen students (50%) had already had PMP training. Regarding the PMP learning session they had just had, the learners had a favourable impression. Ninety per cent of learners felt that the PMP was a useful way of learning that would change their way of thinking. and agreed that it should be used regularly for teaching. Eighty per cent of learners thought that the PMP was better than other means of learning but also considered that the PMP was a reliable means of assessment. 76.6% were in favour of its regular use during SMCEs but 66.6% of learners thought that the PMP was a stressful means of assessment.

Our work had a few weak points, but it nevertheless enabled us to achieve our objectives and propose the following recommendations at faculty level.

- To promote the production and validation of several PMPs within the Nephrology Section and to create a database containing at least two PMPs for each pathology listed in the DCEM2 externship logbook (one for the formative evaluation and the other for the ECOSM).

- Generalise the use of the PMP as a means of learning from the first practical training courses, as part of a well-coded curriculum with well-defined educational objectives and standardised planning across the various training sites.

- Incorporate the PMP into all MSCE tests and clinical examinations.

REFERENCES

1. Tabbane C. Elements of introduction to medical pedagogy workshops. Centre de Publication Universitaire. 2000.

2. McCarthy WH, Gonnella JS. The simulated Patient Management Problem: a technique for evaluating and teaching clinical competence. Br J Med Educ. 1967;1(5):348- 52.

3. Golchai B, Badgaren T, Mojtaba S, Majidi S, Golchi J. Students views about GDM Education with EPMP (Electronic Patient Management Problem) Method Procedia. Social and Bahavioral sciences. 2012; 47:2104-6.

4. Marquis Y, Chaoulli J, Bordage G, Chabot JM, Leclere H. Patient-management problems as a learning tool for the continuing medical education of general practitioners. Med Educ. 1984;18(2):117-24.

5. Yardley S, Dorman T. Kirkpatrick's levels and education evidence. Med Educ. 2012;46:97- 106.

6. Fontaine S, Loye N. l'évaluation des apprentissages : une démarche rigoureuse. P Med. 2017; 18 :189-98.

7. Le Mauff P, Bail P, Gargot F, Garnier F, Guyot H, Honnorat C, Huez JF. L'évaluation des compétences des internes de médecine Générale. Aspects théoriques, réflexions pratiques. Exercer. 2005 ; 73

:69-72.

8. Charlin B, Bordge G, VanDER VLeuten C. Evaluation of clinical reasoning. P Med. 2003 ;4 :42-52.

9. Jouquan J. L'évaluation des étudiants en formation médicale initiale. P Med. 2002 ;3 :38-52.

10. Audetat V, Sandra G, Laurin S. l'évaluation formative, pourquoi et comment? Le médecin du Québec. 2014 ;49 :71- 3.

11. Gilibert D, Gillet T. Revue des modèles en évaluation de formation : approches conceptuelles individuelles et sociales. Pratiques Psychologiques. 2010;(16):217-38.

12. Al-Jasmi F, Moldovan L, Clarke J. Computer-assisted teaching of mucopolysaccharidosis by patient management problems. Mol Genet Metab. 2009;96(2): S12.

13. Biran LA, Biran L, Dunn WR, Harden RM. Using the overhead projector to present patient management problems to groups. Med Teach. 1985;7(3-4):257-69.

14. Yoon BY, Choi T, Choi S, Kim TH, Roh H, Rhee BD, et al. Using standardized patients versus video cases for representing clinical problems in problem-based learning. Korean J Med Educ.

2016;28(2):169-78.

15. Roblyer ND. When is it "good courseware"? Problems in developing standards for micocomputers courseware. Educ Technol. 1981;21(10):47-54.

16. Newble DT, Hoare J, Baxter A. Patient management problems. Tssues of validity. Med Educ. 1982;16(3):137-42.

17. Blewett EL, Kisamore JL. Evaluation of an interactive case-based review session in teaching medical microbiology. BMC Med Educ. 2009;9(56):1-9.

18. Mackenzie CT. Dental student perceptions of case-based educational effectiveness. Journal of Dental Education. 2013;77(6):688-93.

19. Thistlethwaite JE, Davies D, Ekeocha S, Kidd JM, Macdougall C, Matthews P, et al. The effectiveness of case- based learning in health professional education: A BEME systematic review. Med Teach. 2012;34:421-44.

20. Van Stappen Y. The case method. Pédagogie Collégiale. 1989;3(2):16-8.

21. Romainville M, Coggi C. L'évaluation de l'enseignement par les

étudiants: Critical approaches and innovative practices. De Boeck Supérieur; 2009.

22. Afroza S. Use of a PMP manual as a teaching tool to accelerate paediatric teaching in Bangladesh. Med Teach. 2000;22(4):365-9.

23. Ben Abdelaziz R, Hajji H, Boudabous H, Ben chehida A, Mrad-Mazigh S, Azzouz H, Tabib N. Learning Pediatrics through the Patient Management Problem: contribution and perception of students. Tun Med. 2018 ; 96 :1-5.

24. Sedlacek WE, Nattress LW, Jr. A technique for determining the validity of patient management problems. J Med Educ. 1972;47(4):263-6.

25. Page GG, Fielding DW. Performance on PMPs and performance in practice: are they related? J Med Educ. 1980;55(6):529-37.

26. Dillon GF, Clyman SG, Clauser BE, Margolis MJ. The introduction of computer-based case simulations into the United States medical licensing examination. Acad Med. 2002;77(10 Suppl):S94-6.

27. Norcini JJ, Swanson DB, Grosso LJ, Webster GD. Reliability, validity and efficiency of multiple choice question and patient management problem item formats in assessment of clinical competence. Med Educ. 1985;19(3):238-47.

ABSTRACT

Background:

The Patient Management Problem (PMP) is a pedagogical tool that was developed in the mid-1960s in the United States. The aim of this study was to assess the impact of PMP-based learning in practical nephrology education, as well as students perception of the value of PMP in their learning and evaluation.

Methods :

We conducted a prospective evaluative study at the Nephrology Department of Mongi Slim Hospital. We included DCEM2 medical students. We prepared an electronic-format PMP on the management of life- threatening hyperkalemia in chronic hemodialysis patients. The teaching session included a briefing phase, followed by a pre-test, individual completion of the PMP, a debriefing phase, a post-test, and a satisfaction questionnaire.

Results :

Thirty students participated in the study. 83% scored above the passing mark during the PMP evaluation. The PMP significantly improved test scores and thus facilitated the acquisition of new knowledge. This improvement was observed irrespective of the students initial level. Half of the students (50%) had prior experience with PMP-based learning. Regarding the recent PMP learning session, students had a favourable impression. Ninety percent of the students believed that PMP was a useful learning tool that would change their way of thinking, and they agreed to its regular use in teaching. 76.6% were in favour of its regular use in ECOSM (formative assessments), but 66.6% of the learners found that the PMP was a stressful evaluation method.

Conclusions:

PMP is an effective and well-received learning method by students. Its use should be extended to all disciplines for both teaching and assessment purposes.

TABLE OF CONTENTS

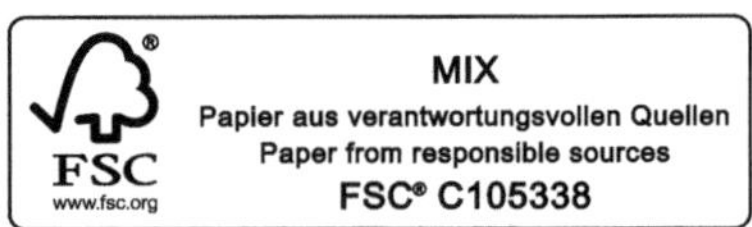

Printed by Books on Demand GmbH, Norderstedt / Germany